Paint a Double Rainbow

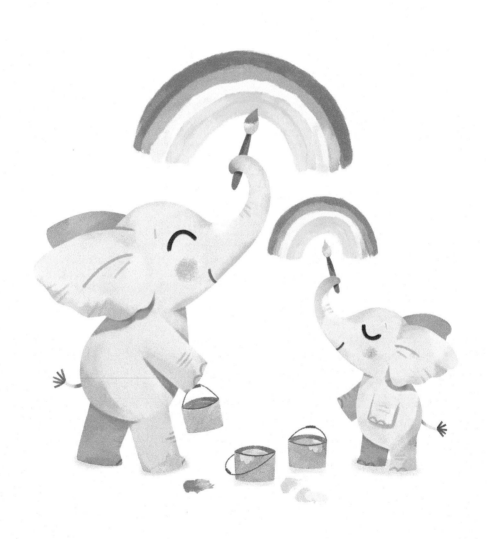

PAINT A DOUBLE RAINBOW

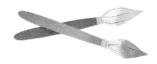

40 MINDFULNESS ACTIVITIES

FOR KIDS AND THEIR GROWN-UPS
TO FEEL CALM, FOCUSED, AND HAPPY

SALLY ARNOLD

Z KIDS · NEW YORK

To my beloved family.
I love you unconditionally,
all the time, truly and forever,
with all my heart.

CONTENTS

MINDFUL
TOGETHER

This little book will transform your parenting in a big way. As a mindfulness educator, nurse, parenting coach, and mom of four children, I teach how mindfulness can change brains to improve focus, decrease stress, alleviate anxiety, and increase curiosity, wonder, and compassion.

Parents often report that they are seeking a deeper connection with their child. They are looking for ways to *be* with their child, rather than adding them to their already too long to-do list. Parents want to slow down and connect with their child in a meaningful way.

The activities in *Paint a Double Rainbow* are invitations to explore mindfulness and experience a heartfelt presence that will bring both joy and a deeper parent-child connection.

In these pages we will explore what mindfulness is and discover fun ways to integrate it into your daily life.

This book is ideal for children ages four through eight. Their minds are curious and imaginative, their hearts are open, and they are learning to navigate big feelings—they're at the perfect age to build a mindful toolbox. After delving into these activities, you may notice your child practicing mindfulness alone, or find yourself taking three mindful breaths when you want to respond instead of react.

A fun way to explain mindfulness to children is to tell them that back in the "olden days" people didn't exercise. They wouldn't just go for a run. They would run only if a bear was chasing them! Since then, science has shown us how important exercise is for the body. Today we have running shoes and races and enjoy regular exercise. Science has also shown us that mindfulness is as good for the brain as exercise is for the body. Let your child know that mindfulness helps us focus, have less stress, feel calmer, and be happier.

The activities in this book are based on neuroscience, intended to enrich the growing brain of the child and to relax the (possibly stressed-out) brain of their grown-up. Each time the activities are practiced, a skill is built, new brain connections are made, and the connection with your child deepens.

It is best to make special time to do these activities, when there are no other distractions. I recommend that you begin with "Breathe Together" to understand the basic breathing practices. The rest of the activities do not need to be done in any particular order. Most of the activities use items that are readily available at home or found in nature (though there are some activities that will require a few inexpensive purchases and a bit of planning). For simplicity, I occasionally refer to "parent" and "child" in this book. However, I encourage any loving adult to enjoy these activities with their child or children.

Just as exercise has long-lasting results for the body, mindfulness has long-lasting results for the mind, and especially for the developing brain. May this book be an inspiration for you and your child to slow down, be fully present, and enjoy meaningful mindful activities together.

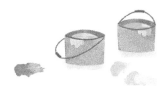

BREATHE
TOGETHER

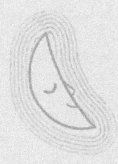

Did you know that your lungs fill and empty over 20,000 times each day? Most of the time you don't pay attention to your breath or your breathing. Noticing your breath and regulating your breathing are simple ways to calm your nervous system.

Breathing is the foundation of mindfulness. This chapter offers activities that build on mindful breathing. Some activities take place outside, some are interactive, and some are for quieter moments. Most importantly, all the activities are meant for exploration and fun.

Take 3

If you are feeling overwhelmed, sad, afraid, stressed, or anxious, Take 3 will help you feel better. Take 3 is the simplest activity in this book and the activity you will both use the most!

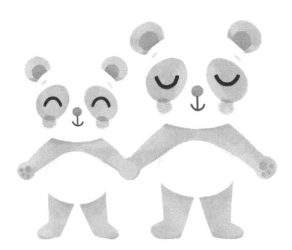

Gently hold each other's hands.

Close your eyes and take three slow,
deep breaths together.

With each breath, place your attention on the air
passing through your nose and down into your belly.

Notice your belly fill like a balloon on the inhale,
as you breathe in.

Notice your belly empty on the exhale,
as you breathe out.

Take 3 is mindful breathing. It is a mindful reset.

You can Take 3 anytime, anywhere.

You can Take 3 with a partner or alone.

Now whenever you see "take three mindful breaths"
in an activity, you'll know how to Take 3!

Breathing
Buddies

This is a great activity for tuck-in time. Enjoy a snuggle and practice with your breathing buddies together.

WHAT YOU'LL NEED:

2 of your favorite Beanie Baby–sized stuffed animals
These are your breathing buddies.

Find a comfy space on the floor or on a bed
where you can lie down next to each other.

Place the breathing buddies on your bellies.

Close your eyes or gaze softly at one spot.

Slowly take in a big breath,
breathing in to the count of three.

Even more slowly,
let out the big breath to the count of five.

Repeat 5–10 rounds with your breathing buddies.

Which breath makes your breathing buddy rise?

Which breath makes it fall?

Share with each other how you feel
after this activity is done.

Animal Breaths

Get your silly on! This breathing activity is fun and interactive. Decide who starts, and then take turns.

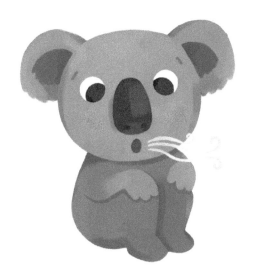

The first person calls out an animal like "Cow!"

Together, take a deep breath in,
then breathe out the sound a cow makes.

Inhale and say "Mooooo" as you exhale.

The second person calls out
a different animal like "Cat!"

Together, take a deep breath in,
then breathe out the sound a cat makes.

Inhale and say "Meoooooowww" as you exhale.

Take turns naming animals and making animal sounds
together all the way through the exhale.

What would a horse breath sound like?
What would a dolphin breath sound like?

Be creative and let the animal sounds be silly and fun!
Start with five animals each.

Star Wands

Make these charming star wands
together to practice mindful breathing.
Keep your star wand by your bed
if you can't sleep or get scared at
night. Breathing together at bedtime
is relaxing for both of you.

WHAT YOU'LL NEED:

2 jumbo pipe cleaners

12 large plastic star beads

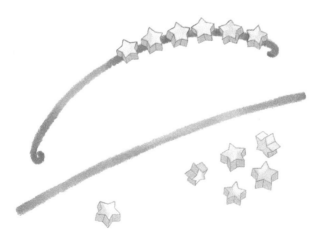

Curl one end of the pipe cleaner
so the beads won't fall off.

Arch the pipe cleaner like a shooting star.

Thread six star beads onto the pipe cleaner.

Curl the other end to hold the beads on.

Find a quiet place where you can sit together.

Begin by gathering all the stars
on the left side of the wand.

Breathe *in* as you slowly shoot one star across the wand.

Breathe *out* as you slowly shoot
another star across the wand.

Repeat until all six stars are
on the right side of the wand.

Want to feel even more relaxed?

Breathe all the stars on the right side back to the left.

On your very last star, make a wish!

Big Bubble Breaths

Add bubbles to your mindful breathing
with this fun-for-two activity.

WHAT YOU'LL NEED:

2 toy bubble bottles with
wands and bubble soap

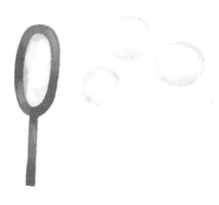

Begin with both of you dipping your wands
in the bubble soap.

Take a slow breath in, and hold your breath
to the count of three.

Softly, slowly, blow bubbles through the wand.

Watch the bubbles as they swirl into the air.

What kind of breath makes more bubbles?
Faster breaths? Slower breaths?

Try sharing your bubble blowing in mindful silence.
This can be a calming experience.

Now make your bubble blowing lively!
One of you tries to pop the other's bubbles and
counts them for recorded points.

In both activities, practice controlling your breath
as you make big bubble breaths.

Finger Breathing

This finger breathing activity has three parts. First, practice finger breathing using your own hand. Second, practice finger breathing with your partner's hand. Third, your partner traces your hand and breathes with you.

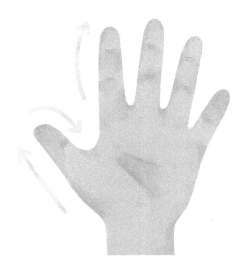

Begin with an open hand, fingers stretched out.

Use your pointer finger from the opposite hand as the tracer.

Begin tracing your hand from the outside base of your thumb.

Breathe *in* through your nose as you trace *up*.

Pause when you reach the top of your thumb.

Breathe *out* through your mouth as you trace *down*.

Trace all five fingers.

How slow can you go? Slow as a snail?

Now use your pointer finger to trace your partner's fingers, breathing together.

Switch and let your partner trace your fingers, breathing together.

How are you both feeling after practicing finger breathing?

Floaty Feather Breathing

Sometimes when you have big feelings, like feeling scared or angry, you hold your breath or breathe really fast. Controlling your breathing is a tool to help you feel calm again. One way to feel calmer is to make your exhale breath longer than your inhale breath. In this activity, you get to practice controlling the exhale breath with a floaty feather.

WHAT YOU'LL NEED:

A feather that fits in your hand (or a leaf)

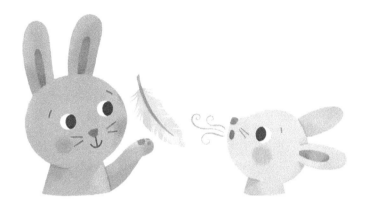

Open your hand, palm side up.
Place a feather on your hand.

Have your partner softly blow the feather
off your hand to the count of five.

(Tip: Aim the breath under the feather.)

What happens if your partner blows too fast?
What happens with short breaths?

Switch and blow the feather off your partner's hand.

Do you feel calmer?

Pocket
Pebble Pal

Mindful breathing helps you regulate
your feelings and decrease your stress.
You will both feel calmer when you hold
your pebble and take mindful breaths.

2 pebbles

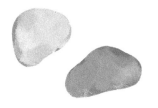

Find two pebbles.
Each of you tucks one into your pocket.

Your pocket pal is a reminder pebble.
It is a reminder to practice your mindful breathing.

If you feel stressed, hold your pebble pal
and take several slow, mindful breaths.

If you feel scared, hold your pebble pal
and take several slow, mindful breaths.

If you have big feelings, hold your pebble pal
and take several slow, mindful breaths.

If you feel alone, remember that
each of you has a pocket pebble pal,
and take several mindful breaths.

You can practice breathing together
or separately. Either way, your pebble pal
makes a good, calming, mindful friend.

STRENGTHEN YOUR SENSES TOGETHER

You are aware of life through your senses: sight, hearing, smell, touch, and taste. Your eyes let you see, your ears help you hear, your nose lets you smell, your skin helps you feel touch, and your mouth (your taste buds) lets you taste.

This chapter offers activities to practice paying attention to your senses, one sense at a time. This focus is called mindful awareness. Noticing your senses, one at a time, helps you bring your attention back into the moment. Practice using your senses of seeing, hearing, smelling, touching, and tasting with these fun activities.

I Spy with My Mindful Eye

In this activity you will strengthen
your sense of sight by getting
your mindful spy eyes on!

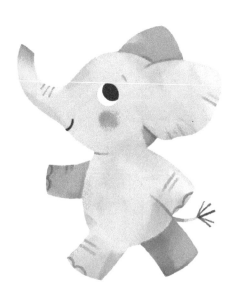

Enjoy a relaxing walk outside together where each of
you picks a color you want to focus on.

Name your color (like red).

As you walk, both of you search for something red.

When one of you notices something red,
say out loud, "I spy with my mindful eye . . .
a *red* wagon!"

Use your spy eyes to search for the first color
for about five minutes.

Switch. Your partner names their color.

Use your spy eyes to find that color.

With older children,
count how many of each color you find.

Keep track to see who has the most mindful spy eyes!

A Silent Sandwich

This activity helps you be more aware of your food and explore your senses at the same time. Start by making the sandwiches together and talking about each ingredient.

WHAT YOU'LL NEED:

Ingredients to make two delicious sandwiches

Silverware for making the sandwiches
and plates for serving them

Where did each ingredient come from?
Imagine the journey of each ingredient to your plate.
Who made this food possible?
Farmers, truck drivers, store employees?

Savor your sandwich in silence, one bite at a time.
Begin to explore your five senses.

What do you **hear**?
Is your tummy grumbling?
Do you hear crunching?

What do you **smell**?
Is it pleasant or unpleasant?

What do you **touch**?
Feel the sandwich between your fingers.
Can you feel different textures?

What do you **see**?
Check out the colors and shapes.

What do you **taste**? Salty? Sweet?

Set your sandwich down between bites.
Pause. Notice. Taste fully.

Stop when you feel full.
Share your experience with your partner.

Hear That
Like a Bat!

Bats fly through the quiet night
using their hearing to find their
way. Like bats, we can hear more
in silence. This activity will help
strengthen your sense of hearing.

This silent sound hunt can be done
sitting outside or going for a walk together.

Use your best bat ears to hunt for
five different kinds of sounds.

Take turns hunting for:

An animal sound
(like dogs barking or birds chirping)

A nature sound
(like the wind or leaves)

A car sound
(like honking or an engine starting)

A voice sound
(near or far)

A soft sound
(like the sound of your heartbeat)

Experiment with sound by
closing your eyes and listening.
Are sounds easier or harder to hear
with your eyes closed?
Try following a sound until it stops.
Where did it go?

Paint a Double Rainbow

One of the most magical parts of sight is your ability to see color. And color goes hand in hand with feelings, which are a big part of mindfulness. Try this activity together to bring more mindfulness to your senses.

WHAT YOU'LL NEED:

1 sheet of paper

2 watercolor paint sets (or colored pencils or crayons)

2 paint brushes

Cup of water to rinse brushes

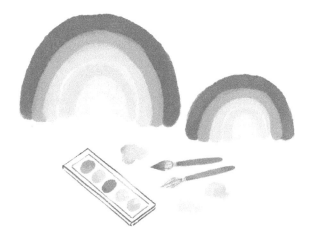

Together, on the *same* piece of paper, each of you paints a rainbow. Then ask yourselves, if feelings were a color, what color would they be? Imagine a feeling that goes with each color of your rainbow.

You and your partner do not need to have the same feeling for each color. Yellow could feel like happiness to one person and scared to another. Only you know how colors feel to you. Your feelings are never wrong. Share the feelings you have for each color with each other.

This creative activity will help you describe big feelings as they arise in the future.

Martian Scientist Tasting Lab

Imagine you are both Martian scientists and you have just arrived from Mars. Your mission is to explore two small, silver-wrapped objects. In the tasting lab (also known as your kitchen), examine the objects. You have *no* idea what they could possibly be!

WHAT YOU'LL NEED:

2 Hershey's Kisses

Investigate your objects, sharing observations with each other, one sense at a time.

Examine your object with your mindful eyes.

Observe the sound of your object
with your mindful ears.

Unwrap your object
with your mindful fingers and touch it.

Detect the odor of your object
with your mindful nose.

Explore the object
in your mindful mouth.
Slooooowly!

Close your eyes and with keen scientific detail notice *all* the sensations.

Share your observations with each other.

To finish your mission, come up with a creative Martian word to name your object.

Say your Martian word three times, and you will suddenly morph back into human form!

Invisible Energy Experiment

Try this activity to feel energy and heat. Can you touch them? Then see what happens when you make a small change in your experiment.

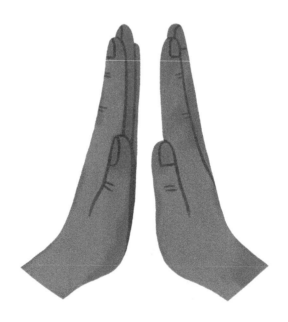

The Invisible Energy Experiment has two parts.

To start, each of you rubs the palms of your hands together to the count of 20. When you reach 20, stop rubbing and keep your palms together.

Ever so slowly, separate your hands until they're about an inch apart. What do you notice? Share your observations with each other.

Now repeat this activity with your eyes closed.

Rub your palms together to the count of 20.

Slowly separate your hands until they're about an inch apart. What do you feel?

Does it feel different from when you kept your eyes open? Why do you think that might be? Was what you felt invisible? Share your experience with each other again.

Stories
in the Sky

This activity uses your sense
of sight plus intentional focus
and lots of creativity.

WHAT YOU'LL NEED:

A sky with fluffy clouds

2 pillows

2 blankets or towels

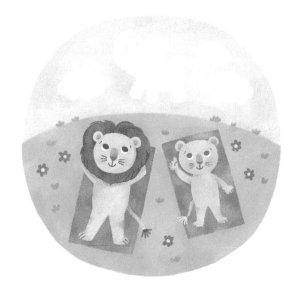

Find a quiet, cozy spot outside.
Lie on your blankets and pillows and create a cloud-gazing story together. We often **look** at the clouds, but we don't always **see** the clouds.

The first person finds an image in the clouds and begins to tell a story about it.

"Once upon a time there was an *elephant* (a cloud) who loved to eat . . ."

(The second person finds the next image)
". . . *broccoli* (a cloud) because broccoli was his favorite food. Then one day . . ."

(The first person continues)
". . . the *boat* (a cloud) collected all the broccoli and the elephant was sad until . . ."

(The second person continues)
". . . a *mouse* (a cloud) brought . . ."

(The first person continues)
". . . more *broccoli* (the cloud) and . . ."

The story goes back and forth, weaving imaginations and clouds, until someone says, "the end."

Tasty Guesses

In this activity the blindfolded
person sharpens their keen
senses of smell and taste.

WHAT YOU'LL NEED:

1 blindfold

6 different kinds of food

Pencil and paper to keep score

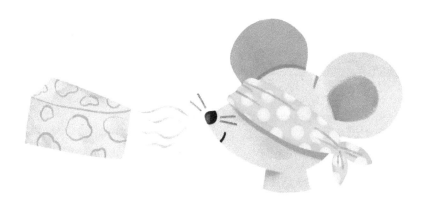

Each person chooses three different
kinds of food from the kitchen.
Keep your food covered so the
other person cannot see it.

Put a blindfold on your partner.

Offer them the secret foods, one at a time.

They try to guess the food by its smell.

If they can't guess the food by its smell,
they try to guess it by its taste.

The blindfolded person tries to guess
what the first three foods are.

Then put a blindfold on yourself and repeat the activity.

If you guess a food by the smell you get two points;
if you guess it by the taste you get one point.

Each person tries to get all three tasty guesses right.

Who had the most tasty guesses points?

FOCUS TOGETHER

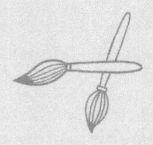

Did a teacher ever tell you to pay attention? Of course! Did anyone ever teach you *how* to pay attention? Most people were just told, never taught. To be able to learn in school and to do jobs as grown-ups, being able to focus is very important. Where we place our attention and knowing how to focus are learned skills. Imagine if a scientist, a teacher, a mechanic, or a nurse couldn't focus. How could they do their job? This chapter is a collection of activities to playfully practice mindful focus.

Can You Breathe with Your Feet?

Since feet don't have a nose or a mouth,
we don't *really* breathe with our feet!
But we can breathe as we walk, pairing
each step with each breath. This
activity will enrich your focus as you
balance your steps with your breath.

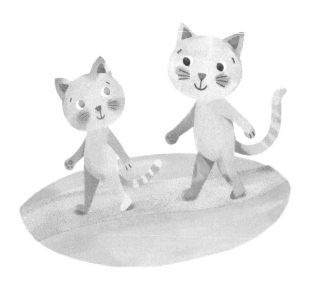

Find a flat area outside where both of you
can walk 10 paces in silence.

Begin at one end of your path.
Start with three mindful breaths.
Walk very slowly together,
imagining that your breath is tied to your foot.

When you breathe **in**, lift your foot **up**.

When you breathe **out**, place your foot **down**.

Take 10 steps, walking heel to toe,
breathing with your feet on each step.

With each step you can repeat in your mind:
"in . . . up" and *"out . . . down."*

At the end of your path, turn around and go back.

Walk your path three times.

How do your feet feel?

Was it hard or easy to breathe with your feet?

Share with each other what you noticed.

MIMEfulness:
Up, Down,
All Around

Partners bring their focus and attention
to becoming *mimeful* as they copy
this pattern at the same time.

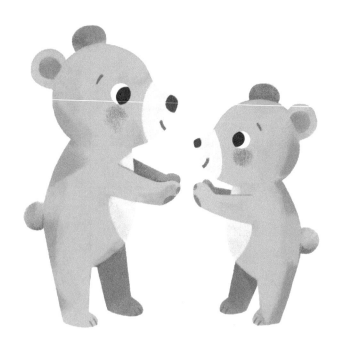

Begin in a standing position.
Imagine that you are both silent mimes.
Face each other with your hands at shoulder level,
palms toward each other, about five inches apart.

Take three mindful breaths together.

Bring your focus to your hands.
Both of you slowly move your hands in this pattern:
up, down, all around.

Move your hands *up* while breathing *in*
to the count of three.

Move your hands back *down* to the center point,
breathing *out* to the count of three.

From the center point, move your hands in a complete
circle (about the size of a steering wheel), breathing *in*
and *out* as you make the all-around pattern.

Practice the up, down, all-around pattern several times.

Then have fun creating your own patterns
with one of you as the mime leader and
the other one as the mime follower.

Still Chillin'

Stillness practice grows peacefulness. Beginning a stillness practice can feel wiggly and squirmy. Your mind might be busy. That's OK. Each time you chill in stillness, finding your anchor (your breath) gets easier. When life feels big and wobbly, you can find your breath and feel peaceful inside. Returning your focus to your breath is key to this practice.

WHAT YOU'LL NEED:

2 yoga mats (or towels)

A stopwatch

A quiet place to sit

Set your mats side by side.

Once you're both settled, start the stopwatch.
Close your eyes and put your hand softly on your belly.
Take three mindful breaths.

Feel your anchor (your breath in your belly).

Keep your attention on your breath.

Notice your thoughts as they pop into your head.
Gently bring your focus back to your breath.

Feel the rise and fall of your belly.

Continue focusing on your breath.

Notice the time on the stopwatch when you're done.

How long did you each practice Still Chillin'?

One minute of stillness is an excellent start!

Ready, Aim, Breathe!

This activity uses focused breathing
to play a fun game for two.

WHAT YOU'LL NEED:

2 Solo-sized cups

2 straws

6 ping-pong balls (or cotton balls)

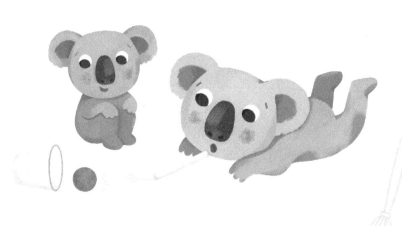

Each of you gets three ping-pong balls to aim and
breathe into the cup.

Both of you lie on the floor,
on your bellies, holding a straw.
(This activity can also be done sitting at a table.)

Place the cup on its side about an arm's distance away,
the opening facing you.

Place the ping-pong ball near the end of the straw.

Take a big inhale and slowly exhale through the straw.

Aim the ball into the cup.

Stay laser-focused with your breath control
to get the ball into the cup.

How many breaths did it take?
Who got their three balls into the cup first?

Mirror Dancing

This activity practices fun, laser-focused
dancing. Have fun being mindful of
your moves and your partner's moves.

WHAT YOU'LL NEED:

Your favorite upbeat music

If you dance while looking in the mirror,
your reflection dances with you.
Your reflection makes the exact same moves you make.

Mirror dancing is a mindfulness
dance party for two! One person is the dancer
and the other person is the mirror.

Find a space where you can move freely.

Decide which person is the dancer
and which is the mirror.

Turn up the tunes and get your groove on!

The dancer rocks out while the mirror follows
with the exact same moves.

After one song, switch off playing dancer and mirror.

Left, Right, Squeezy Tight!

This activity requires focus to decide
on which body part to tighten, relax,
and then to completely release.

Lie down and take three mindful breaths together.
Close your eyes.

Imagine you are both relaxing on a cloud.

The first person calls out a body part (like eyes).

Breathe in and hold your breath
while you squeeze that body part.

Squeeze the left eye, then the right eye, squeezy tight!

Let out a big breath and relax both eyes.

The other person calls out the next body part
(like hands).

Breathe in and hold your breath.

Squeeze the left hand, then the right hand,
squeezy tight!

Let out a big breath and relax both hands.

Play Left, Right, Squeezy Tight until you have
tightened and relaxed as many body parts
as you can call out together.

Feel yourselves fully relaxed. . . . *ahhhh!*

BE KIND TOGETHER

Imagine if your friend broke their arm on the playground. When you try to imagine what they are feeling, that is called empathy. When they come back to school in a cast and you hope they feel better soon, that is called compassion. If you make them a get-well card, or carry their backpack, that is called an act of kindness. Compassion, empathy, and kindness are learned skills. Practicing these skills helps your brain grow and you can become more mindful of those around you. The activities in this chapter will help you get your *mindful kindful* on!

Kindness Catcher!

Kindness is a superpower. It can increase happiness, decrease stress, and build connections with others. Here's how to mindfully catch acts of kindness together.

WHAT YOU'LL NEED:

A shoe box (or small box) with a lid

Markers or colored pencils and stickers

Precut slips of paper

Pen

Have fun decorating a shoe box together.
This is your kindness box.

Make a slit in the lid (to slide notes through).

Keep the box, papers, and a pen in a central place.

Set out your kindness box at the beginning of the week.

Talk about acts of kindness.
Acts of kindness include being helpful,
patient, generous, thoughtful, and caring.
Even a smile is an act of kindness!

Catch each other in an act of kindness.
Write each kindness you caught on a slip
of paper and tuck it into your kindness box.
No peeking until the week is over!

At the end of the week, make a special time to
read all the acts of kindness together.

How does it feel to give and receive kindness?

Celebrate all the acts of kindness with a big hug!

Secret Kindness Club

Did you hear about the secret kindness club? Members of this special club practice secret acts of kindness. You'll both use mindful awareness to plan this activity.

THESE ARE THE CLUB RULES:

1. Do something kind.

2. Keep it a secret.

Start a secret kindness club with your partner.
Plan an act of kindness and don't get caught!

Here are some secret kindness ideas
you can do together:

Help an older person carry their groceries.

Make thank-you cards and take them
to a local police or fire station.

Bake cookies and drop them off (in secret)
to someone who is having a hard time.

Visit a nursing home,
even if you don't know anyone there.

Have fun thinking of creative ideas
to practice secret acts of kindness.

Oh, and thanks.
The secret kindness club makes
our world a better place!

Rock On!

Try to imagine what someone might
be feeling (empathy) and paint a rock
that might cheer them up (compassion).
Have fun painting kind words and
cheery pictures on rocks together
and then tucking them in places for
people to find: a bus stop, a park
bench, a grocery basket, a café table, a
doorstep. Discovering a kind rock will
delight the person who receives it!

WHAT YOU'LL NEED:
Paint brushes
Acrylic paint
Multi-surface paint pens
Smooth, flat rocks

Gather your rocks. Wash and dry them.

Paint one side with acrylic paint. Let it dry.

Write your word with paint pens
or draw a picture on your rock.

Inspirational words include
Smile . . . Joy . . . Peace . . . Breathe . . . Love . . . Be Kind . . .
Happiness . . . Just Be . . . Sparkle . . . Thankful . . .
Blessed . . . Shine . . . Believe . . . Courage . . . Gratitude . . .
Laugh . . . Remember . . . Mindful . . . Hope . . . Grace

Pictures ideas include a heart,
a peace sign, clouds, a happy face.

Have fun tucking your kind word rocks in secret places!

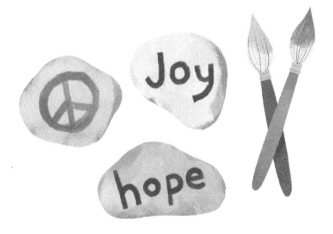

Sending Kind Wishes

Sending kind wishes is like sending an emotional text. We can send kind wishes to anyone: family members, friends, people who need extra love (maybe kids who are not kind at school), and even ourselves. This activity can be done alone or with each other.

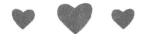

Begin with three mindful breaths.

Think about someone who needs kind wishes.
Imagine them doing something they enjoy.

With your eyes closed,
place your hands over your heart.

Fill your heart up with a bubble of love.

This bubble will carry three kind wishes.

As you imagine sending your bubble of love,
say these wishes out loud:

May you be happy.

May you be healthy and strong.

May you be filled with peace.

Imagine the person smiling back at you as they receive
the kind wishes sent from your bubble of love.

How did it feel to send kind wishes?

Moonlight Gratitudes

Moonlight gratitudes is a special time to share with each other the moments that filled your heart with gratitude. At bedtime, snuggled close, talk about how gratitude is the feeling of appreciation: appreciation of things big and small, appreciation of simple moments and ordinary experiences. You can feel grateful for the extra special things too.

Take three mindful breaths together.

Think about your day,
and recall three things
that made you feel grateful.

Share the first thing
you are each thankful for,
followed by a mindful breath.

Share the next thing
you are each thankful for,
followed by a mindful breath.

Share one thing you are thankful for
about each other,
followed by a mindful breath.

Tuck in with a kiss, a hug,
and a wish for sweet dreams!

IMAGINE TOGETHER

Your brain can't tell if something is real or imaginary. Try to remember a time when you felt scared. Maybe you were scared at night because you thought you saw a monster in your room. When you turned on the light, the monster disappeared. Even if the monster wasn't real, those scared feelings felt big inside your body. Practicing mindfulness helps you pause and notice what you're thinking and how you're feeling.

You can choose where to place your thoughts, to imagine things that make you happy. When you focus on happy moments, you will feel good. The more you practice thinking about things that feel good, the more positive pathways you build in your brain, and the happier you feel.

I Am! I Am! I Am!

Saying your *I ams* in front of a mirror
is a powerful mindfulness practice.
How you speak to yourself makes
a difference in how you feel about
yourself. Use your imagination to see
yourself as the best version of you.
Speak your *I ams* out loud and begin to
see yourself as you truly are. Which
three words celebrate the best of you?

WHAT YOU'LL NEED:

A mirror

Together, stand in front of a mirror.

Place your hands over your heart.

Feel the warmth and tenderness.

Take three mindful breaths together.

Recite your *I am*s out loud, one person at a time.

"I am ... *strong!*"

"I am ... *kind!*"

"I am ... *love!*"

Finish your *I am*s with one big mindful breath.

You can also use your star wand
(see page 12) to practice your *I am*s.

Here are a few words to get you started.

I am
Healthy ... Funny ... Happy ... Peaceful ...
Courageous ... Light ... Joyful ... Whole ... Brave ...
Capable ... Creative ... Generous ... Worthy ...
Friendly ... Curious ... Gentle ... Caring ... Bright ...
Honest ... Confident ... Silly ... Magnificent ...
Thankful ... Compassionate ... Kind

Imagine a World . . .

Enjoy this activity side by side, sitting or lying down. Tell a story about an imaginary world where everyone feels happy, safe, and peaceful. This world can be realistic, fantasy, or silly. Take turns telling the story, sentence by sentence.

Focus on details, such as the senses (see, hear, smell, touch, taste) as you go back and forth telling your story. When you imagine with your senses, your positive feelings become stronger. Make this epic world feel great!

Imagine a World is a wonderful way to meet a new day and a sweet part of tuck-in time at night. It is also a happy way to pass a long car ride.

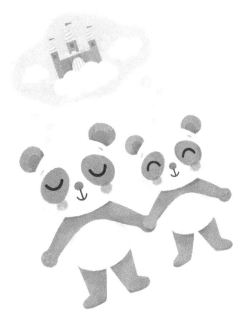

Start your story with "Once upon a time there was a world where . . ." and include details like:

Trees have edible chocolate leaves.

Kids can fly to their friends' houses.

Birds sit outside your window and sing you to sleep.

Raindrops fall in shimmery rainbow colors.

Everybody is safe, all the time.

Big Feeling Bubbles

We all have worries and stresses and big feelings (scared, sad, anxious, angry). Did you know that your brain can decrease a feeling just by naming that feeling? In this activity, you both name a big feeling you want to release.

WHAT YOU'LL NEED:

2 toy bubble bottles with wands

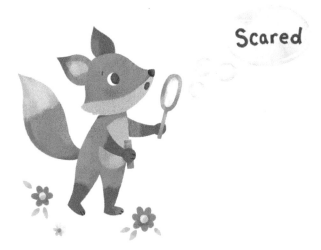

Scared

Begin by taking three mindful breaths together.

Name the big feeling you want to release.

As you each blow through a wand, imagine blowing
your big feeling into the bubbles.

The biggest bubble will be the one
to hold your big feeling.

The big feeling bubble will carry your feeling away.
Watch the bubble until it pops or disappears.

Want to let go of more feelings?

Keep playing with your big feeling bubbles!

Give Me a Dream

Use your imagination to give a
dream at bedtime, and make this
ritual the heart of your day.

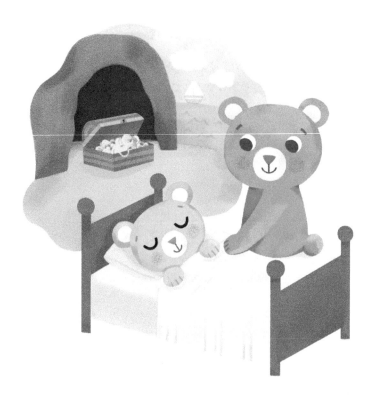

The dream giver needs two details
from the dreamer: a name and an object.

For example:

Dream giver:
"Once upon a time there was a little boy named . . ."

Dreamer: "Alex."

Dream giver:
"One day Alex was hiking into a deep
dark cave where he found a . . ."

Dreamer: "secret treasure box."

The dream giver makes up the story of
Alex and the Secret Treasure Box. When the story
gets close to the end, the dream giver tenderly
hands the story over to the dreamer by saying:
"Now it's time to finish this story in dreamland."

Give the dreamer a gentle hug
and let them float off to dreamland.

Sweet dreams!

Sunshine Grounding Cord

When you have big, overwhelming feelings (anxiety, sadness, fear), you need to stop and reset. This activity helps you slow down and come back into the moment.

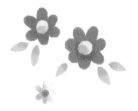

Find a spot where you both can stand outside, barefoot, in the sunshine. (You can also do this activity on a blustery day, inside, barefoot, using even more of your imagination.)

Stand side by side with your eyes closed.
Take three mindful breaths together.

Imagine tiny roots growing from the bottom of your feet, deep, deep into the earth.

Take three mindful breaths.

Feel the warm sun on your face.

Imagine a big cord of shimmery sunshine pouring into you from the top of your head through your body and down into the earth.

Take three mindful breaths.

Feel the light inside.

Feel the roots growing.

Feel your breath.

Now you are grounded with the earth and the sky.

Happy Memory Mini Movie

Fun fact: Your brain can't tell if something is actually happening right now or if your thoughts are from a memory. This activity focuses on a happy memory and grows good feelings. What we focus on grows.

Each of you chooses a memory of
one of the happiest times of your life.

Watch this memory as if it's a
mini movie playing in your mind.

Watch your happy memory mini movie
for about three minutes.

Notice the details. The more details you
remember, the happier you will feel.

Bring your senses into your mini movie.

Who was there?   What did you hear?

What did you see?   What did you taste?

What did you smell?   What did you touch?

How did you feel?

When your movies are over,
sit or lie side by side in mindful silence.

Take three mindful breaths.

Share your experiences with each other.

What was the best part of your happy
memory mini movie?

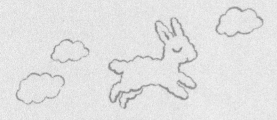

RELAX TOGETHER

We are human *beings*, not human *doings*. But sometimes we get caught on the hamster wheel of life. Going and going, doing and doing, forgetting how important it is to slow down. This chapter is an invitation to make time to relax and just *be* together. It gives you activities that support calm minds and calm bodies. Each activity brings you back into this moment. This moment is where the best of life lives. Enjoy relaxing together!

Heel to Toe: How Slow Can You Go?

Massage combines touch, connection, and relaxation—and a foot massage can relax your whole body.

WHAT YOU'LL NEED:

Lotion

A towel

2 pairs of socks

Soft music

Start playing the music.

Take three mindful breaths together.

Let the grown-up take the lead.

Tuck the towel under your child's clean feet.
Warm the lotion (about the size of a quarter)
in your hands by rubbing them together.

Massage the first foot slowly from the heel to the toe,
adding more lotion when needed. Ask "Is the pressure
good? Too light? Too firm? Just right?"

Rub the bottom of the foot to the top of the foot,
and around each toe. Massage the second
foot the same way. How slow can you go?
Can you massage as slow as a sloth?

Remind your child to find their breath,
to feel the rise and fall of their belly.

Trade foot massages with each other,
doing 5–10 minutes per person,
until you're both relaxed.

Put socks on those happy feet when you're done!

Magical Traveling Healing Light

This body scan activity combines relaxation, connection, and imagination. One person is the guide and the other is the traveler.

A blanket to lie on

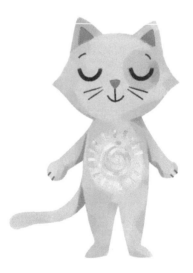

Lie down together and take three breaths.

The guide tells the story of a magical healing light that travels through the traveler's body. This light starts at the top of their head and slowly moves to their toes.

The guide tells the traveler where the light is shining in their body, then pauses, giving the traveler time to move their attention to that body part.

As the guide speaks, the traveler imagines the magical healing light traveling inside their body, shining relaxation and healing into each part.

The guide reminds the traveler to take deep breaths as they focus on each part of their body.

If you're the traveler, notice how peaceful you feel after the light travels through your body. What color was your light?

Take turns being the guide and the traveler.

Peace Corner

A peace corner is a special place where you can be still and feel peaceful, either alone or with each other. (Try to keep the space uncluttered, and never use it as a punishment or time-out corner.) Here's how to create a relaxing peace corner in your home.

WHAT YOU'LL NEED:

A rug to define the space

A small table

2 floor pillows

Colored pencils and paper

A nature basket with found items like shells, acorns, pine cones, smooth pebbles, feathers, and leaves

A star wand (see page 12)

A calm jar (see page 94)

Breathing buddies (see page 8)

Talk with each other about how you
want to use your peace corner.

It can be your special place to practice stillness.
It can be a quiet place to be with your thoughts.
This can be your place to unplug from the
busyness of the world and to recharge.

In your peace corner you can relax
with your calm jar or star wand.

What other activities from this book
could you do in your peace corner?

Try Big Feeling Bubbles (see page 72),
Floaty Feather Breathing (see page 18),
and Rock On! (see page 60).

Chalk Walk

Labyrinths have been used for over 4,000 years for meditation and relaxation. Walking a traditional labyrinth is a journey to the center and back out again. Here's how to create your own chalk walk.

WHAT YOU'LL NEED:

Sidewalk chalk

A paved area for drawing

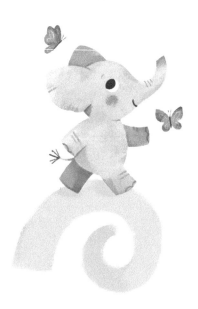

Using sidewalk chalk on a flat surface, draw your labyrinth together. Draw a circle or spiral for a simple design or create your own labyrinth shape.

Think of a word that describes how you want to feel. Share your feeling word with each other.

Choose who goes first.

Let's say you want to feel calm.

As you start walking, following your chalk lines, think "I **feel**" and breathe in.

Think "**calm**" and breathe out.

Repeat your word and your breathing as you walk your labyrinth. Try to stay with your feeling word for the whole chalk walk. When you notice a thought, gently bring your attention back to your feeling word.

How do you feel when you are done?

Let your partner take a turn and then share your feelings with each other.

Safe and Sound

This activity will help you feel safe and sound at any time. Practice it when you are scared or worried or simply want to relax. It will bring attention back into your body and promote a sense of calm and safety. Practice this activity with your partner until you can recite the safe and sound verse from memory.

Standing or sitting,
feel both of your feet on the ground.

Take three mindful breaths.

Place your hands over your heart.

Close your eyes.

Say these words out loud or in your mind:

I feel safe

I feel sound

I feel my feet

on the ground.

Repeat these words at least three times.

Finish with a few mindful breaths.

Did you feel the warmth of your hands over your heart?

When will you use Safe and Sound?
Share your thoughts with your partner.

The Secret
Tiny Pause

Here is a secret just for you! There are
two tiny pauses tucked between each
breath. One tiny pause is tucked between
the *in* breath and the *out* breath. The
other tiny pause is tucked between the
out breath and the *in* breath. Placing
your attention on the tiny pause will
help you feel more relaxed. In this
activity, you'll both find the tiny pause.

Find a quiet place to practice stillness together
(maybe in your peace corner).

Take three breaths.
Feel the rise and fall of your belly.

Breathe in. Bring your attention
to the tiny pause of the *in* breath.

Did you find it?
It's the pause right before you breathe out!

After you breathe *out,* look for another tiny pause.
Did you find that one too?

Spend a minute or two in stillness,
placing your attention on both tiny pauses.

Your Very Own Calm Jar

A calm jar will help you settle down, refocus, and relax. A calm jar is like your mind: when your mind is busy, the glitter spins and swirls. When you breathe mindfully, your mind settles, just like the glitter. Here's how you can make a calm jar together.

WHAT YOU'LL NEED:

1 medium-sized mixing bowl

1 half pint Mason jar with top

¾ cup hot water

¼ cup corn syrup

1–2 drops of food coloring (optional)

1–2 teaspoons of fine glitter (can mix colors)

3 drops of dish soap

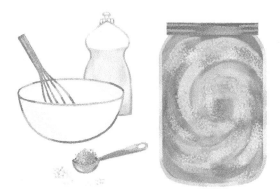

Whisk the hot water and the corn syrup in a mixing bowl.
Pour the mixture into the Mason jar.

Add the food coloring to the jar.
Put on the lid and shake the jar.

Add the glitter. If you're using multiple colors,
use half a teaspoon of each color.

Add three drops of dish soap.

Fill the jar with additional hot water to the top, tighten
the lid, and shake the jar.

To use your calm jar: Shake your jar and set it on the
table. Watch the sparkles swirl. As you practice mindful
breathing, watch the sparkles settle until all the sparkles
are resting at the bottom of the jar.

Feel your body and mind settle too.

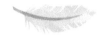

CONCLUSION

I wrote *Paint a Double Rainbow* for small humans and their grown-ups to unplug, practice mindfulness, and recharge together. Would you expect your devices to keep going without being recharged? We too must recharge.

By practicing the activities in this book, you have learned to recharge. You have also created a mindful toolbox. Each activity is a tool, and these tools help you build a more harmonious and peaceful life. The more you practice these activities, the more benefits you will receive, so revisit the activities on a regular basis, alone and together.

My wish is for all children, everywhere, to be blessed by a supportive adult who will explore mindfulness with them. I hope you both continue on your mindfulness path with your new tools and skills, and that you continue to reap all the benefits mindfulness offers.

MORE ABOUT MINDFULNESS

Books

Everyday Blessings: The Inner Work of Mindful Parenting. Myla and Jon Kabat-Zinn.

Myla and Jon Kabat-Zinn are the pillars of mindful parenting. This book is filled with heartfelt wisdom. If you are seeking loving guidance and insight from seasoned parents, you will enjoy *Everyday Blessings.*

Mindful Parenting. Kristen Race, PhD.

Dr. Kristen Race gets real with how hard parenting can be; in fact, she identifies the plight of busy families as "Generation Stress." This book offers relevant life tools to navigate parenting mindfully. You will learn to stress less and connect more.

The Whole-Brain Child. Daniel Siegel, MD, and Tina Payne Bryson, PhD.

This book helps parents understand the brain development of their children. When parents understand basic brain development, they can parent with greater ease and raise happy, healthy, and calmer children. *The Whole-Brain Child* offers tools to address day-to-day struggles with successful resolution.

Self-Compassion. Kristen Neff, PhD.

This is not a mindful parenting book. However, this book deserves to be read by all parents. As parents, we are a surrogate nervous system for our children. *Self-Compassion* reminds us to treat ourselves the way we would treat a dear friend. It helps us be our best self, enriching our capacity to parent from a place of love.

Parenting with Presence. Susan Stiffelman, MFT.

Susan Stiffelman offers empathy, compassion, and guidance for parents seeking support in raising confident, compassionate, and conscious kids. She honors children as "our greatest teachers" and honors parents with tools to parent with greater awareness.

Mindful Discipline. Shauna Shapiro, PhD, and Chris White, MD.

Mindfulness is the foundation of conscious parenting. Parenting requires boundaries and discipline. From setting limits with love to working with difficult emotions, this is a go-to book for practicing mindful discipline.

Growing Up Mindful. Christopher Willard, PsyD.

Here are essential practices to help children, teens, and families find balance, calm, and resilience. Christopher Willard offers practical ways to introduce mindfulness to children and their parents. This book teaches clear, precise practices intended to weave mindfulness into your family life.

Peaceful Parent, Happy Kids. Dr. Laura Markham.

This book teaches you how to be the best version of yourself as a parent. It offers advice tailored to all ages and stages of childhood.

Websites

ahaparenting.com

This website has something for everyone. Dr. Laura offers online classes, taken by over 10,000 parents, as well as books, articles, videos, and podcasts filled with real-life parenting wisdom.

astillquietplace.com

Dr. Amy Saltzman teaches how to access our Still Quiet Place. She says, "A Still Quiet Place is a place of peace and happiness that is alive inside of each person." Dr. Saltzman brings exceptional mindfulness training to children and adolescents, athletes, coaches, and parents. Her website includes videos for practice, online courses, blogs, and links to her mindfulness books.

mindful.org

This website is a wealth of information on all things mindful. From information on brain science to meditation practices, articles about parents, kids, the workplace, relationships, and health, research, and so much more, this website is relevant, science-based, and infused with heart.

mindfulcompass.com

Sally Arnold offers mindfulness tools, teachings, and tips for bringing mindfulness into your daily life. Explore her three flagship programs—The Awakened Parent, Workplace Wellness, and School-Based Mindfulness—and learn about her courses, coaching, and resources created to support you on your mindfulness journey.

susanstiffelman.com

Susan is revered for teaching techniques to reduce power struggles and to stay in charge from a place of love and compassion. Her website includes courses, a podcast, coaching, a blog, and a parenting community.

Apps

Calm

This app offers free meditations or a paid subscription. *Calm* is known for its meditations to reduce stress and improve sleep. The Calm Classroom Initiative offers every teacher in the world free access to *Calm* to empower teachers and their students.

Headspace

This app has a lot to offer. From its podcast to its blog, videos to audio meditations, it offers meditations for mindful parenting. Headspace is excellent for beginners, as well as seasoned meditators.

Stop, Breathe & Think Kids

This meditation and mindfulness app for kids includes mindful activities for 15 situations, sleep stories, video animations, and stickers to celebrate progress. It's a great resource for kids to learn to process and navigate emotions, and it includes interactive child–parent activities.

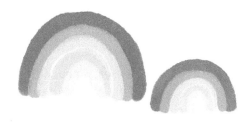

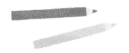

ACKNOWLEDGMENTS

To my students: I am humbled to share mindfulness with you. Thank you for all the lessons you have taught me. You have authored this book as much as I have. These are *our* activities.

Dearest teachers: Thank you for showing up for your students in tireless, selfless, and loving ways. Thank you for inviting me into your classrooms and making mindfulness a priority. I am honored to share this path with each of you.

Meg Ilasco: This book began with your call answering my call. You have been an inspiration to work with; you have made this entire process enjoyable. My deepest appreciation.

Susan Randol: Your desire to bring mindfulness to kids and their grown-ups is visionary. Your exceptional editing translated the work of my heart into this book. My sincerest gratitude.

The Zeitgeist team: I am deeply grateful for this opportunity. It has been a wonderful learning process.

Chris Makena and Megan Cowan: The yearlong mindfulness program with you at Mindful Schools changed the course of my life. Teaching mindfulness to children and parents has been my most rewarding work. Thank you for being my beloved teachers and dear friends.

To my family—Michael, Kelsea, Karl, Alex, Kiana, Kenzie, Quinlea and Aviana: You are my greatest mindfulness teachers. Thank you for your endless support and unconditional love.

ABOUT THE AUTHOR

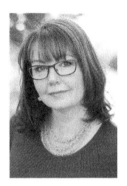

Sally Arnold is an international mindfulness educator, speaker, author, and parenting coach. She holds a bachelor of science in nursing and a master's degree in psychology, and has extensive training in mindfulness education. She is the founder of Mindful Compass, an organization that offers courses designed for families, corporations, and general audiences. Sally has taught mindfulness to thousands of children and implemented whole school mindfulness programs.

Sally and her husband have four wonderful children. Together they have been foster parents and adoptive parents, and have been known to bring home kids who just need a bed, a family, and a safe place. When not writing or teaching, Sally can be found puttering in her garden, hiking in the Sierra Foothills, or reading to her twin granddaughters. Discover more about her and Mindful Compass at *mindfulcompass.com.*

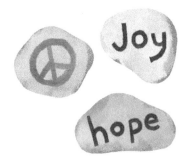